T0349099

SWEDISH
LAGOM

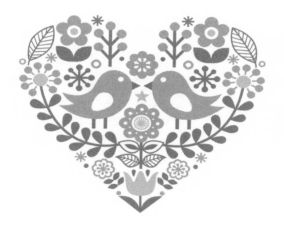

SWEDISH LAGOM

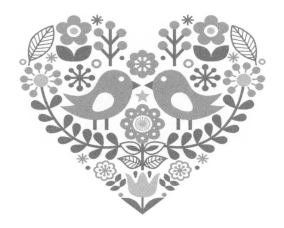

FINDING JOY
IN JUST ENOUGH

Kortney Yasenka
& Karen Johnson Yasenka

Hatherleigh Press is committed to preserving and protecting the natural resources of the earth. Environmentally responsible and sustainable practices are embraced within the company's mission statement.

Visit us at www.hatherleighpress.com.

Swedish Lagom

Library of Congress Cataloging-in-Publication Data is available.
ISBN: 978-1-961293-19-9

Printed in the United States
10 9 8 7 6 5 4 3 2 1

Kortney: For my mother, Karen, and father, David. Thank you for creating a family life filled with unconditional love, cherished memories, and countless family traditions.

Karen: For my granddaughters, Helena and Isla, who will carry on our family traditions of togetherness for years to come.

Contents

• •

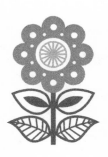

Välkommen

Fear less, hope more; eat less, chew
more; whine less, breathe more; talk
less, say more; hate less, love more;
and all good things are yours.

—Swedish proverb

Year after year, Sweden continues to rank high on the list of the happiest countries in the world. One of the main reasons for this is the uniquely balanced lifestyle of its people. The Swedes even have a name for this concept of balance: *lagom*.

The Swedish word *lagom* literally translates to "just the right amount." Just the right amount of work, just the right amount of relaxation, just the right amount of friends, family and hobbies—finding just the right balance is the secret to a happy life. To feel balanced is to feel in control, which decreases stress and anxiety and increases mindfulness and appreciation.

Fortunately, you don't have to be born a Swede to experience the benefits of a balanced Swedish lifestyle. While there are many factors that go into a *lagom* lifestyle, the basic concept remains the same: embrace balance to find happiness. Although those two little words may seem impossible to achieve, they are actually quite obtainable. If you yourself practice a *lagom* lifestyle and incorporate *lagom* into your everyday activities, it will be easier to pass down a balanced and happy life to your friends and family. After all, a balanced, happy life definitely makes time spent together easier and more enjoyable.

The wonderful secret about finding joy in just enough is that anyone can enjoy the Swedish lifestyle. Living a life filled with *lagom* can easily translate to any cultural background, varying socioeconomic status, different living and relationship statuses, and ever-changing family dynamics.

Lagom living is about finding enjoyment in the little things in life. It means embracing everything that nature has to offer while surrounding yourself with loved ones in a cozy environment.

Many of the Swedish concepts, lifestyle habits, and traditions that contribute to _lagom_ can be adapted to fit any family, and provide a helpful roadmap in the pursuit of personal balance. As the ultimate goal of Swedish living is finding balance, embracing Swedish culture, concepts, and mindsets will naturally lead you to develop your own sense of balance.

That being said, living _lagom_ requires more than adopting a few Swedish habits or following some simple Swedish "life hacks." The Swedish lifestyle also involves creating and maintaining those traditions of the past deemed essential to future happiness. By celebrating and honoring these traditions, passed along from generation to generation, we benefit from a sense of belonging and connection—a sense which has been linked to stronger mental well-being.

Likewise, having your family participate in these traditions year after year strengthens bonds and reminds everyone that we are part of something greater. This, in turn, provides feelings of security, safety, and support.

In addition to a sense of belonging and connection, incorporating traditions into your family's life also provides structure and familiarity. Structure and familiarity offer reassurance during times of stress and uncertainty. The predictability of celebration, tradition and togetherness helps us find peace, balance, and serenity in the knowledge that even as the world changes, the things we hold dearest remain with us. Engaging your family in traditions is also an effective way to create powerful, lasting memories that will be passed down to future generations. Reminiscing about family traditions brings about feelings of nostalgia, which research suggests is linked to happiness and improved mood.

Close relationships, which are a result of strong family traditions, are also linked to increased happiness.[1] Humans are inherently social creatures and close relationships are vital to our overall well-being. Swedish traditions connect current family members to each other, as well as with past and future generations. Swedes understand the impact that traditions and family time have on their quality of life, so the Swedish style of togetherness time emphasizes the importance of simply being together.

Throughout this book, my Swedish mother and I cover many aspects of the Swedish lifestyle, viewed from the perspective of creating long-lasting traditions that help bind you and your loved ones together in a common feeling of balance and togetherness. From home decor to holiday traditions, family recipes and healthy living habits, our aim is to help you and your family become a *lagom* family—the true secret to living a *lagom* life. We by no means claim to be experts in all things Swedish, but my mother is 100 percent Swedish, so she knows a few things! By sharing our family traditions with you, drawn from a multi-generational perspective, we serve as living proof to demonstrate how traditions can be altered throughout the years to best fit your family. Our hope is that you use this book as a resource to help you and your family find balance.

The main takeaway from this book should be the creation of meaningful, lasting, and consistent family time for you and your loved ones. Choose the traditions and aspects of living a *lagom* life that you like best and incorporate them into your life. Alter other traditions to best fit you and your current lifestyle. It was very fitting that while writing this book, my mother and I were able to do exactly what we hope now to convey to you, the reader: enjoyment of time spent together while creating long-lasting memories. I consider myself very fortunate to have written this book with my Swedish mother.

"Happiness is a Swedish sunset it is there for all, but most of us look the other way and lose it."

—MARK TWAIN

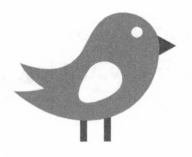

Why Lagom?

Ingen ko på isen.

—Swedish proverb, translated as,
"There's no cow on the ice."
Meaning: Don't worry.

Why is living *lagom* so important? What's really so special about finding joy in just enough?

As a licensed clinical mental health counselor, I am profoundly aware of the number of individuals who struggle to find balance in life and create a meaningful existence. Often times, individuals report feeling a lack of control in their lives; chief complaints during sessions center around clients feeling as though every aspect of their life is suffering because of this imbalance and lack of control. They report feeling as though they don't have enough time for family, or to complete work assignments; they lack the energy to participate in interests and hobbies, and to simply enjoy life. Each day feels as though it melts into the next, stuck on an endless cycle of repetitive motions. Perhaps you feel the same way: as though you are going through the motions, not fully present in your own life, or the lives of your loved ones.

This feeling of imbalance leads to increased anxiety and stress, a longing for a sense of self, a lack of purpose, and it contributes to the development of unhealthy habits. The Swedes determined long ago that this was no way to live life. Life should be purposeful, filled with joy, and experienced alongside family and friends.

Embracing everything *lagom* has to offer and making it a goal to live a *lagom* lifestyle (both you and your family) will have a significant impact on your overall well-being, level of happiness, and cohesion as a family unit. The positive benefits of living the Swedish lifestyle are plentiful and without a doubt the secret to Sweden's success in the realm of personal fulfillment, satisfaction and happiness. Feeling in control, socially connected to others, and a sense of belonging are key ingredients for your mental well-being—and fundamental aspects of living *lagom.*

Lagom and Happiness

I would argue the goal in life is to be "happy." Feeling pleasure, enjoyment, and being content and confident with yourself, your family, your work, and your health, should be what you strive to achieve. A sense of happiness is what leads to better overall well-being, a sense of purpose, belonging, and balance.

The Oxford Language dictionary defines being "happy" as 1) feeling or showing pleasure or contentment and 2) having a sense of confidence in or satisfaction with (a person, arrangement, or situation). Research surveys have also identified specific areas of life that give people the greatest amount of "happiness." These areas are mental and physical health, a sense of purpose, and family connection. (Other factors impacting "happiness" are reported to be living conditions, feeling in control, and spending time in nature.)

For the Swedes, having balance in life is what creates the conditions necessary to achieve all these prerequisites for happiness. Having balance promotes healthy living, both physically and mentally. It helps you manage your time, your energy, and your stress level. *Lagom* allows you to enjoy what makes you happy which leads to a feeling of fulfillment. The carefully designed *lagom* lifestyle allows time for work, family, friends, hobbies, volunteering, exercising, spending time in nature, and relaxing. All these things add to your overall positive mental (and physical) health.

The definition of what it means to be happy can be different for everyone. What makes you happy may be very different from what makes someone else happy. The great thing about *lagom* and the art of Swedish living is the fact that it can be different for everyone. It's about finding the balance that works for you.

For some, this might mean spending the majority of your time with family. For others, it might mean balancing family time and alone time. There's nothing wrong with a *lagom* lifestyle that incorporates "me" time. *Lagom* living can involve cozy nights spent reading alone by the fire, enjoying the company of a good glass of wine while watching your favorite show, or going for a solo hike in the woods. Finding a little bit of solitude each day may be the perfect *lagom* lifestyle for you.

There is a saying in Sweden: *lagom är bäst*, which translates to, "*Lagom* is best." This little phrase certainly sums up the art of Swedish living: simple, purposeful, and to the point. Since *lagom* can be used as a noun, adverb, adjective, and even a verb, I propose incorporating *"lagom health"* as a new phrase and way of life—not just for Swedes, but for everyone! Imagine if everyone adopted this way of living. Everyone would experience a newfound sense of mental and physical health. *Lagom* represents a way of living optimized for the challenges of the fast-paced modern world, providing a restored sense of belonging through a self-care routine incorporating healthy habits, traditions, social connections, and resilience—all qualities that everyone would find useful and beneficial.

Everyone wants to live a fulfilled, successful, and meaningful life: one filled with laughter, happiness, and connection. Living *lagom* and practicing finding joy in just enough can bring you and your family one step closer to finding balance.

The Swedish Family

Familjen är inte en viktig sak. Den är allt.

—Swedish proverb

Meaning: Family is not an important thing.

It's everything.

How it all began, as told by my mother, Karen:

In 1948, a young seventeen-year-old girl left her hometown of Avesta in the province of Darlana, Sweden. She voyaged aboard the USS Stockholm to start a new life in America. Her name was Birgit Maria Persson, my mother. In 1950, she married Ivar Carl Johnson, a second-generation Swede whose parents, Emma and Theorin, had immigrated to America from Varmland, Sweden in the late 1800s. It is because of their union that Swedish traditions have been celebrated and passed down through five generations, from my grandparents to my parents, from my parents to me, from me to my children, and now from my children to my granddaughters.

Growing up in a Swedish household, I Kortney, was exposed to a Nordic lifestyle filled with family traditions. As a child, I didn't think much of how my parents did things. This was especially true with regard to my mother (as she is 100 percent Swedish) and her mother, my *mormor* (which translates to mother's mother in the Swedish language), who was born and raised in Sweden. But the more I learned about the traditions and mindsets specific to Scandinavian countries, the more I realized that these philosophies were naturally embedded into my life.

Spending time together is an integral part of living like a Swede. The Scandinavian lifestyle focuses on appreciating and enjoying experiences, with family time being a big focus. That being said, while the time spent together *should* be quality time, *quantity* of togetherness time is also, if not more, important. The family unit is strong in Swedish culture, but the term family is open to interpretation as the Swedish culture is more accepting of all types of families. For example, it is not uncommon for Swedes to forego marriage but still have long, committed relationships and children. In fact, most Swedes will not get married until they have children with their partner. Despite this (and in fact because of it), mutual respect, autonomy, and uncon-ditional love are core values of the Swedish family.

Valuing togetherness and putting in the effort to create family time signals to your family mem-bers that they are loved. Swedes know the power of family time and encourage it from an early age. Children are seen as equals and mutually respected; there is no mindset of "children should be seen and not heard." Swedish families gladly welcome child-led discussions and child-led activities. It's no wonder that Sweden was the first country in the world to explicitly prohibit all forms of corporal punishment and other means of punitive treatment of children.

The practices and philosophies important to Swedish families remove the separation between parent and child. There is no need to have a "kids table" for holidays or separate television-watching before bed; togetherness for Swedes means being a family unit where everyone feels valued and where everyone knows their opinion, views, and input matters.

Spending time as a family also undoes the notion that your child matters less simply because he/she is a child. The Swedish way is to incorporate your child in most, if not all, family things. By doing so, you create an expectation that, because you include your child in your activities, discussions, hobbies, etc., your child will gladly and willingly choose to include you in *their* life both now, and going forward into the future. This level of connection and togetherness time spans far past childhood for most Swedish families. It's very common for adult children to spend holidays with parents, vacation with parents, and meet up for weekly dinners.

The other secret to the Swedish style of spending quality time together is that it doesn't need to take the form of extravagantly planned outings. Of course, vacations, holidays, and "big" events are exciting and filled with lifelong memories, but the best and most impactful quality times are those little day-to-day moments you spend with your family. It's the times before bed, the family breakfasts, the helping with school projects and household tasks, and the time spent just in each other's company. Sometimes, the most lasting memories of togetherness are when you are "just there" for your family.

The act of just simply being there for your family allows you to gain a deeper understanding of your family members. Being there, at all times, creates consistency and reliability—two key concepts in *lagom*, as we discussed previously. Being present, mindful, and free from distraction allows you to fully experience and enjoy togetherness time.

In our family, we take every opportunity to share in each other's accomplishments and interests. We attend all musical recitals, athletic games and competitions, school performances, open mic nights, etc. We all support each other's interests all the time! Time goes by so quickly and we don't want to waste a minute of it!

If you weren't born into a close-knit family, or if you have chosen to disassociate with your family for good reason, you can still find benefits to living the *lagom* lifestyle and incorporating Swedish living techniques into your own life. Friends are said to be the family life chooses for us, so adopt the *lagom* lifestyle into your interactions with your support group, whomever that may include.

The Lagom Lifestyle

In this chapter, we'll look at some simple starting strategies that will help you live the *lagom* lifestyle, just like a Swede.

Rise and Shine
Becoming a Morning Person

Morgonstund har guld i mund.
—Swedish proverb, translated as,
"Morning hour has gold in its mouth."
Meaning: Wake up early; those
hours are the best.

The best way to begin living a more *lagom* lifestyle is to start first thing in the morning! Each day should be started early and with a purpose in mind. The phrase "sleeping in" was, and still is, not in my vocabulary. The feeling of getting up before sunrise and watching the new day begin is awe-inspiring. There is something very calming, motivating, and energizing about watching the sun come up.

Seeing the start of each day as a new beginning, a fresh start, and a brand-new opportunity will allow your brain to stay focused, optimistic, happy, and well-balanced. If you begin each day with this mindset, not only will you start things off on the right foot but so will your family! You will be modeling healthy, pleasant ways to begin the day for the other members of your family.

Believe it or not, taking advantage of the morning hours may also make you a happier person. According to research conducted at the University of Toronto, people who wake up early tend to feel happier than those who stay up later. Early rising gives your brain the mental boost it needs to be more alert and productive throughout the day. Feeling this way will also give you a higher level of patience which will create more positive interactions and togetherness time with every member of your family, and yourself.

Not to mention, rising early allows for more time in the day. With so many people reporting a constant feeling of time crunch, as though there aren't enough hours in the day to get everything done, having a few extra hours first thing in the morning makes you more able to enjoy moments and practice patience. Swedes value punctuality and allowing for ample time in the morning is a way to ensure they are never late.

This could not be any truer for my mom! To this day, I can without a doubt say my mother has never been late to anything. Her ability to always be on time is some type of Swedish superpower. My father, on the other hand, as Swedish as he would like to be, was not born with this trait. Another reason why my mother and father are the perfect balance (or, should I say, perfect *lagom*) for each other.

Each morning my mother would make me and my sister and brother breakfast before school. We would come downstairs, the table would be set, and we would sit in our "assigned seats." (I don't know if the Swedes can claim this habit as a cultural mainstay, but for some reason we always sat in the same seats around the kitchen table.) While not quite what I would call a family tradition, it definitely provided a sense of security, familiarity, and consistency. My mother would have our lunches packed (with a note, of course) and ready to go for us.

Allowing for more time in the morning also gives you and your family the ability to spend time together in a calm and relaxing manner before the busy day begins. Talking about what the day had in store for each of us helped us prepare and plan for the hours ahead. We packed our school bags, gave lots of hugs and kisses, and hopped into our father's car. We were lucky enough that our father had a flexible work schedule and was always able to drive us to school. Car rides to and from school (where our mother would pick us up) made for a wonderful way to add togetherness time and find that balance during a hectic day.

If you are feeling as though becoming an early riser is not something that will come naturally or easily to you, here are some tips and strategies that will help you and your family enjoy early mornings together:

Change your perspective of what being a morning person means. Rather than dreading early mornings, view it as a time for you and your family to mentally prepare for the day and focus on the upcoming opportunities. Swedes hold the optimistic view that each day marks a new beginning filled with new possibilities. Use positive self-talk to help change your perspective. Instead of saying you *have* to get up early, say to yourself you are *able* to wake up early. View it as a privilege, not a punishment.

Transform the bedrooms in your house to have gradual light shine in during the early hours. This will be easier to do during the summer months.

During the colder and darker winter months, add soothing lights and candles to your room to ease your morning wake-up. A gradual increase from dark to light will make the transition feel more natural.

Try to get outside and into nature as quickly as you can. Go for a walk, a run, or a bike ride. If your schedule doesn't allow you to spend a significant time outside in the morning, try just opening your window or stepping outside for a few moments while enjoying your morning coffee. Being exposed to the outdoors first thing in the morning has numerous benefits to your physical and mental health.

Place your alarm clock or phone on the other side of the bedroom. If the physical act of getting out of bed is the most difficult part for you, this makes it so you have to actually get out of bed to turn off your alarm. As with any new behavior, it will take some time before becoming a habit. If you are having trouble with getting up earlier, give it some time and most importantly, remind yourself of the benefits of being an early riser for you and your loved ones.

Embracing the Outdoors

Det finns inget dåligt väder,
bara dåliga kläder.

—Swedish proverb, translated as, "There is
no bad weather, there are only bad clothes."
Meaning: Prepare for situations and make
the best out of external conditions.

I'm almost certain that every child has heard their parents or grandparents say, "When I was young, I had to walk to school, uphill, both ways, in the snow." To this day, when I hear this phrase or something similar to it, it always brings a smile to my face along with a quiet chuckle. I'm not laughing because of the ridiculous exaggeration; I am laughing because in my case, it was true.

Ever since I was young, I vividly remember my *mormor* telling us stories about how she would have to ski to school in Sweden. She would tell us of the days when she was younger, how *everyone* skied to school, or to the store, or to go to a friend's house. My *mormor* would throw her backpack over her shoulders, click into her cross-country skis, and make the trek to and from school every day…and yes, some of it actually *was* uphill.

British author, Alfred Wainwright, inspired by a Swedish proverb, wrote: "There's no such thing as bad weather, only unsuitable clothing." He certainly had the right idea when it comes to embracing the outdoors and experiencing all that nature has to offer. His philosophy on weather conditions and the outdoors is without a doubt ingrained into the Swedish culture and way of living.

Ecotherapy, also called nature therapy, is defined as a group of techniques or treatments using nature to improve mental or physical health. Developed by Theodore Roszak as a subpart of the emergent field of ecopsychology, he believed that having a deeper connection to nature can improve your interpersonal relationships and emotional well-being.

Swedes wholeheartedly believe in the positive impact nature can have in your life and on your overall sense of wellness, because of the way nature helps you find balance. (That said, my mother often says that a Swede's love of the outdoors and embracing the harsh winter weather was for some reason not passed down to her. As Swedish as my mother is, she is not one to spend hours outside in the woods, especially in the colder months. She would much rather enjoy a cozy room with dim lighting, and warmth you can actually feel!)

Not only is ecotherapy said to have lasting

positive effects, but it can also be a memorable bonding experience. Time in nature is another excellent way to spend togetherness time with your family. For Swedes, this isn't anything out of the ordinary; they probably don't even realize they are practicing ecotherapy. I'm almost certain that, were you to ask, they would just say they like being outdoors. It's a way of life for many Swedes.

Fun Fact: It's a common practice in Sweden to have babies and infants nap outside. Preparation is key, and of course they are dressed appropriately for the weather conditions. Many Swedish parents, and researchers, have found that this practice of sleeping in the outdoors increases the quality and quantity of sleep. This Swedish parenting routine exposes children to the wonderful and plentiful benefits of nature at a very early age. This makes it easier to continue to spend time in nature even when children get older. What a wonderful tradition and practice to instill in your children, one that can and will be passed down to generations to come.

Learning to embrace the outdoors, no matter what the weather may be, demonstrates determination, persistence, perseverance, and most importantly, the ability to make the most out of any situation. These are all qualities most Swedes possess that help increase their level of *lagom*. I was fortunate enough to have strong role models of persistent Swedish women in my life. My *mormor's* life story, which we briefly recounted earlier, was one of true resilience. Leaving her family and home country of Sweden when she was just seventeen years old and immigrating to the United States, all while being unable to speak English, strongly demonstrates these Swedish qualities. Her ability to accept these circumstances (though she did not have much choice in the matter) also showcases her traditional Stoic mindset and an ability to make the best out of a situation that is outside of her control.

Emotional Regulation

Spending time in nature is also said to help strengthen emotional regulation. Simply put, emotional regulation is the ability to manage and exert control over your emotions.[2]

It's a common misconception that Swedes are emotionless. Swedes have emotions and express them, but Swedes don't let their emotions control them. In all my life with my *mormor*, I only saw her cry once. It was in the hospital when my *morfar* (grandfather) died.

Now, I am by no means saying crying or show-ing emotion is wrong in any way, but my *mormor's* ability to regulate her emotions even in a time of grief was impressive. She felt her emotions, but she didn't let them control her. I know how much my *mormor* loved my *morfar*—they were married for 60 years—and I know she was extremely shocked and saddened over his sudden death, but she was still able to maintain her composure and think rationally.

Growing up, my family was and still is extremely affectionate and loving. Everyone who knows us always comments on how close we are and how much time we spend together. Some people even find it a little odd. For myself, I still can't understand why people think spending time with your family is strange. I consider my siblings my best friends and spend most of my time with my family. We say "I love you" all the time and we all know and appreciate how much we care for one another.

Because I am mostly Swedish (as well as a little British and Slovak, thanks to my dad), being in control of my emotions is literally in my DNA. Although we are an extremely affectionate, close, and loving family, we don't let our emotions get the better of us. Everyone in my family is very stoic, even-tempered, and rational. I believe (and scientific study supports) that time spent in nature at an early age helps build strong emotional regulation skills. The ability to regulate your mood and emotions increases your ability to effectively collaborate and communicate with others.[3]

By choosing to focus on the positives in your situation, you are actively creating memorable and fun experiences for both you and your family. Togetherness time in nature lets you turn a rainstorm into puddle jumping and rainbow chasing. It allows you to enjoy an impromptu snowball fight; it creates togetherness time while relaxing in a hammock under the summer sun.

My siblings and I like to say we grew up "in the woods." We were fortunate enough to have about an acre or so of wooded property right in our backyard. In my naivety as a child, I assumed everyone had woods in their backyard. I never understood why people went camping. I thought, "Can't they just go in their backyard?" I now realize that I was extremely fortunate and that my parents, when moving from Connecticut to New Hampshire, specifically chose a building lot with an abundance of nature and woods. My mother has even said that the birch trees sprinkled throughout our backyard reminded her of the birch trees in Sweden.

These woods kept us busy for hours on end. We would play "house" in the woods with everyone having their own little piece of land, complete with a rock we pretended was the bed and a stump we used for the kitchen table. This free play in the woods allowed us to be creative and develop an entire world of make believe and pretend games. The family joke now is that my siblings and I always say my mother would "make" us go outside and play. As if we weren't allowed inside to play! My siblings and I are very grateful for this now, as my childhood memories are filled with outside adventures and togetherness time with my family. This is something that has been passed down to my nieces, Helena and Isla, and hopefully on to their children as well.

Spending time in nature and immersing yourself and your family in the full experience not only connects you to nature but can also give you a feeling of awe. Experiencing more awe is associated with living a healthier and more meaningful life and is correlated with feeling lower levels of stress.[4] Awe-inspiring moments change how you perceive the world and yourself. Incorporating experiences that give you and your family the feeling of awe is yet another way to enjoy your togetherness time and find balance.

Appreciating time in nature with your family not only connects you to the great outdoors and gives you a feeling of awe; it also boosts your mood. Outdoor time encourages free play, which improves your focus, and helps you and your family develop executive functioning skills while building confidence, and increasing your level of gratitude and appreciation.

It goes without saying that spending time outdoors also increases your overall physical activity level. Being physically active has tremendous positive effects on your mental health.[5] Add exercise with outdoor time, and you've doubled your benefits! Adhering to the philosophy of embracing the outdoors also pairs well with being an early riser. Studies have shown that being exposed to sunlight first thing in the morning profoundly affects your mood. According to research, exposure to full spectrum sunlight in the morning increases serotonin, which helps us sleep better at night, and improves your mood throughout the day.[6]

If you are looking for ways to engage in more time spent outdoors with your family, try some of the following:

- Go for a hike

- Watch a beautiful sunrise or sunset

- Travel to new places

- Stargaze at night

- Experience live entertainment or sporting events together

Remember, the main goal of togetherness time is to spend time with your loved ones. It's about bonding, connecting, listening, validating, and experiencing moments together. These moments don't need to be expensive or extravagant adventures. It's about making the most of any situation and focusing on the positive aspects of everything you do with your family. Walks to local parks, community gardens, playgrounds, and public pools and beaches are other ways to spend time in nature, even if you live in a more metropolitan setting. You can even find many activities right in your backyard that are completely free. Spending time in nature will benefit your whole family and by doing so you may even feel more balanced and happier: the goal of *lagom* living.

By accepting and welcoming every weather condition, you are showing yourself and your family that you will not let circumstances change what you had planned while also focusing on the positives rather than the negatives of a given situation. This type of mindset allows you to make the most out of your togetherness time.

The many benefits of spending time in nature can be realized with family and friends, or by yourself. Creating *lagom* lifestyle habits early on will help you incorporate them into your future family life, if you choose that path.

Having trouble embracing the outdoors? Here are some easy ways to approach a more nature-friendly lifestyle.

Start doing "normal" things outside. Incorporating the outdoors into your daily routine will make it easier for this *lagom* practice to become a lifestyle change. You could start by taking phone calls outside, setting up an outdoor office, and eating meals outside.

Make your outdoor space inviting. Whether you have many sprawling acres as your backyard or an outside living area that can barely fit a chair let alone a table, spending more time outdoors is possible. The whole idea of *lagom* is finding just the right amount. You don't need an excessive amount of space to enjoy the outdoors. Set up a small chair or table, decorate with a few lanterns or candles, and have a cozy throw blanket nearby to help you enjoy outdoor living anytime of the year.

Take your hobbies outdoors. Spending time in nature is known to increase levels of creativity.[7] What better way to get your creative juices flowing while also reaping the benefits of being in nature? Whatever your hobby or interest may be, try engaging in it while outside. If you don't currently have any ongoing hobbies, this is a great time to start. Painting, writing, knitting, woodworking, gardening, or reading, the list is endless.

Green exercise. The term green exercise refers to any physical activity that is done outdoors. This strategy combines nature and working out which has double the benefits. If you don't currently engage in physical activity, make an effort to go for a walk, run, hike, or bike outside.

If you are already a lover of fitness, change up your routine to incorporate more green exercise.

Know the benefits. To help motivate you to spend more time outdoors, educate yourself on the many benefits of ecotherapy. This can be done by reading books, watching documentaries, or researching different nature-based interventions.

Give it time. Keep in mind that incorporating nature and outdoor living into your life can be a gradual process. Invest in appropriate weather-related gear and apparel to make the most of your experience. Spending time in nature can actually become somewhat addictive, but in a positive way. The more time you spend exposed to the outdoors, the more time your body and mind will want to spend outside.

Community Involvement

Wherever you turn, you can find
someone who needs you. Even if
it is a little thing, do something for
which there is no pay but the privilege
of doing it. Remember, you don't
live in the world all of your own.

—Astrid Lindgren, Swedish author

Det är lyckligare att ge än att motta.

—Swedish proverb

Meaning: It is happier to give than to receive.

The Swedes have a concept called *Jantelagen*,
which translates to "the Law of Jante." According
to many Swedes, it is the basic belief that no one
is better than anyone else. Your focus should be
on doing good and Swedes hold the mindset

that everyone, no matter who they are or what they do, is equal and should be treated as such. This concept emphasizes collectiveness and a sense of togetherness, all while working for a greater good.

Ever since I can remember, my family and I have always been involved in some form of community outreach. My father, being a Lutheran minister, created countless programs through his church that helped not only his congregation but also the community as a whole. (We came to the conclusion that my father was really a social worker disguised as an ordained Lutheran minister.)

I have memories of visiting the local nursing home and socializing with the residents, collecting Christmas gifts for families in need, stocking shelves in the church's food pantry, eating lunch with adults with varying difficulties in our church's fellowship hall, and doing annual spring yard clean-up for individuals not able to do so on their own. My childhood was filled with helping others; however, it wasn't something that was talked about in great depth. My parents didn't recite research on the benefits of helping others or even really tell us the importance of what we were doing. It was just something that was part of our daily life.

My father was not born a Swede, but he definitely lives like one. Directly after retiring from the ministry, my father started a local non-profit that assists the housing insecure and unhoused population in our area. My father saw a need in our community and through his hard work and dedication, an embodiment of *Jantelagen* called Isaiah 58 NH was created.

Over the past ten years, Isaiah 58 NH has become a stable resource for community members in need of services and resources. Seeing the difference my father makes in his community gives me hope, inspiration, and motivation that I can do the same. This is the type of mindset you should aim to pass down through the generations to come. The Swedes certainly know how to make the gift of giving a generational habit—a habit that helps not only those in need, but the helpers, too.

The Gift of Giving

The term "Helper's High" was first coined by Allan Luks in his book, *The Healing Power of Doing Good* to describe the positive feeling people have after volunteering. Doing something kind for someone else promotes a prolonged feeling of calmness, a reduction in stress, and a greater sense of self-worth. These positive feelings have a direct result on how you interact with others. The more positive feelings you experience, the more positive interactions you will have with others. Being involved in the community and volunteering your time to help others will make togetherness time with your family more mean-ingful and enjoyable. Creating family traditions such as charity involvement will strengthen your family unit and have a direct positive result on yourself and others—a wonderful *lagom* life, filled with balance.

Being philanthropic, altruistic, and involved in your community also has positive effects on your mental health. There are countless studies showing that acts of altruism are strongly correlated with the "feel good" chemicals in your brain. According to the Cleveland Clinic, helping others and being involved in your community and charity work can lower blood pressure, increase your self-esteem, decrease levels of depression and stress, and can even make you live a longer life with greater happiness.

Feeling connected to your community or cause—anything aimed at promoting the greater good—has been proven to improve your overall well-being. And what has *lagom* shown us? If you are in good overall health, then so is your family. Positive role modeling and a positive outlook towards your community while being mindful of how you can assist others will without a doubt be passed down to other family members.

Creating positive life experiences during your togetherness time is a core value of the Swedish family. Engaging in activities that make you and your family feel like a part of something will lead to more feelings of *lagom* by connecting you to family members through a shared bonding experience. It not only models a healthy and happy lifestyle; it also provides you the opportunity to spend meaningful and memorable times with loved ones outside your immediate family.

Becoming more involved in your community may seem like a daunting task, so here are a few strategies to help you get started on your journey:

Pick your passion. Figuring out what type of organization you want to get involved with is the first step. Choose an area that interests you. For example, it could be supporting children, animals, unhoused individuals, the elderly population, or nature conservation. This will help you decide how you want to spend your time.

Get local. Look to your own community first and see what non-profits are in your area. Research local charities and get familiar with their mission statements and philosophy. Then make a call or send an email inquiring about possible volunteer opportunities.

Set a goal. Determine how much time you can devote to your community involvement and set a goal for yourself. Any amount of time helping others is a good use of time. Find the right amount that fits into your schedule. This can be anywhere from once a week to a few times a year.

Delad glädje är dubbel glädje; delad sorg är halverad sorg.

"SHARED JOY IS A DOUBLE JOY;
SHARED SORROW IS HALF A SORROW."

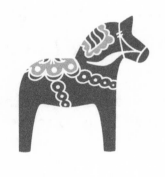

The
Swedish Home

Borta bra, men hemma bäst.

—Swedish proverb translated as,
"Away is good, but home is best."
Meaning: Home sweet home.

I will forever remember all the Swedish items my mom incorporated into our home. The first that comes to mind, something that none of my other friends had in their homes, is the Dala Horse.

My childhood is filled with memories of many Dala Horses in my *mormor's* (as well as my parent's) home. Beautifully painted handmade wooden horses, the Dala Horses we had (and there were many) were mostly red ones with a few blue—horses of all different sizes. We had Dala Horses on everything, from table runners and serving trays with the Dala Horse embroidered and painted on it to Dala Horse jewelry, all made in my *mormor's* hometown of Avesta, located in the Dalarna region of Sweden.

The Dala Horse is more than just a household decoration: it is one of Sweden's oldest symbols and represents qualities such as strength, wisdom, faithfulness, and dignity. These are the same qualities I see in my most favorite Swede, my mother. A strong, wise, and dignified woman, I often thought my mother was ahead of her time when it came to equality for women. My mother wrote the code of ethics for our town, fought tirelessly for school improvements when she was chairperson of the school board, and was involved in local and statewide politics. Leading by example, my Swedish mother instilled the idea that women were equals and that our views and opinions mattered. My father wholeheartedly believed the same, and so my parents raised us to embody these views. I believe this is one of the best gifts parents can give their daughters.

When I began doing more "official" research while writing this book, I had many a-ha! moments. What I had thought of as "just my parents' way of doing things," I quickly learned were actually longstanding Swedish traditions and customs. Sweden upholds the belief that equality is a constitutional norm, and their aim is for women and men to have the same opportunities, rights, and responsibilities in all areas of life. This is evident in a lot of Sweden's governmental policies and is yet another example of *lagom* living and balance. Thank you, Sweden!

Your home is where you and your family typically spend most of your time together. Given the choice, wouldn't you want that space to be inviting, calming, relaxing, and free of clutter? My *mormor* and mother are both extremely neat and organized individuals. My *mormor's* house was very minimalistic, never a thing out of place. My parent's house is very similar; granted, they have more possessions, but you would be hard-pressed to find any dust on the tables or dishes left in the sink. My mother vacuums daily (often twice a day), dusts daily, cleans her sink with Comet every night, and applies special stovetop cleaner nightly. There are no crumbs to be found inside her oven or near the toaster.

My mother is known for cleaning before people come over, after people leave, and every time in between. And just as the house was always free of dirt and clutter, it was never lacking in coziness and comfort. My mother kept the house clean in order to make sure it was always warm and inviting.

How does this contribute to living *lagom*? When your environment is well-balanced, your brain will also be well-balanced. There is an abundance of research that explains how the space around you affects your mental and even your physical health. There is a very common saying: "A cluttered space creates a cluttered mind." These words could not be truer for Swedes!

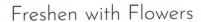

Freshen with Flowers

Walk into my mother's kitchen and you will be sure to see fresh flowers on the table. It doesn't matter what the weather's like or the season—fresh flowers are a staple in my mother's kitchen decor. This preference was something even my mother didn't realize was common to Swedes; when I asked her about it, she told me she just liked flowers. Little did she know it was her Swedish heritage influencing her home decor!

Studies have found that fresh flowers in the home reduce levels of stress, anxiety, and depression.[8] Make it a habit to have fresh flowers in your house to help your family live a more *lagom* life.

Studies have proven time and time again that clutter and disorganization can negatively impact your brain, leading to increased feelings of anxiety and depression and an inability to focus.[9] Sleeping in a cluttered bedroom has also been known to cause sleep problems. Sleep, as many know, is very important, not only for you but also for your family. Create a positive example for your family by having your home free from clutter (or as clear as you can manage). This will help you spend more time together and less time worrying and feeling overwhelmed by your disorganized space.

Döstädning

"A loved one wished to inherit nice things
from you. Not all things from you."

—Margareta Magnusson, Swedish author

Döstädning, the concept known as "Swedish
death cleaning," is more than just simply deep
cleaning your house. It entails rethinking your
relationship with material items and clearing
out space in both your closet and your mind. It
fosters the minimalistic mindset of "less is more."
It's about appreciating what you do have and *not*
focusing on what you don't.

Swedish death cleaning is seen as a selfless
act that puts family first. The idea behind this
tradition focuses on eliminating or cleaning out
personal items from your home before you die, so
that when you *do* die, family members won't be

responsible for the burden. This may seem a little morbid at first; however, when you take the time to think about it, you cannot deny it's very helpful for family members.

While my father is not Swedish by blood, he definitely organizes like a Swede. Our family attic growing up (and still to this day) looks like an ad for IKEA's storage and organizational bins. Complete with printed labels, my father has a bin for everything. Items *are* very easy to find...with the help of a visual map my dad created showing where everything is located. We often joke about how organized and neat my dad is, but boy is it helpful when you're looking for your summer shoes, winter hat, or that trophy from high school!

Maintaining a clean and uncluttered area allows your mind to focus on the more important matters in life and allows you to spend more time together with your family. It also affords you a

comfortable area in which to spend that togetherness time.

Incorporating the Swedish concepts of organization and efficient use of space into your
family's life is about more than creating room
for activities. It's also about creating a certain
atmosphere. Adhering to these traditions and
incorporating them into your way of life will help
create a more balanced, happier, and thoughtful
relationship with your family—increasing your
lagom.

The Swedish home is more about creating a
certain atmosphere of *lagom* than material items.
Finding balance, coziness, strength, and meaning
in your keepsakes is the goal in Swedish living.
Find something in your home or childhood that
brings back fond memories or an item in your
home now that can be passed down to future
generations. In my case, it's the Dala Horse, but
it can be anything that represents you and your
family.

Move Over, Hygge
Mys on the Rise

You may be familiar with the now very popular Danish term "*hygge*." Recently, *hygge* has become a buzzword that has influenced everything from home decor to overall lifestyle. According to the Danes, *hygge* refers to an atmosphere of coziness, comfort, and contentment. Swedes, however, have another term that basically means the same thing. *Mys* is the Swedish word that translates to "cozy," but it is so much more than that. In fact, embracing *mys* is a way of life for Swedes (and for everyone else who wants to live like the Swedish)!

The best way to describe *mys* is that cozy, comforting, and warm feeling you get from spending relaxing time with your loved ones. It's the feeling of contentment, safety, and hominess. It's about relaxing and enjoying the simple pleasures in life. It's about sharing time with loved ones and being in the moment. It's about creating a space for you and your family that is free of stress.

Clearly, incorporating the philosophy of *mys* into your way of life is a great way to spend togetherness time with your family. Embracing *mys* can help you bond with your family while appreciating each other's company. By subscribing to this Swedish way of life, you will not only increase your own happiness but also your family's happiness. These philosophies will, without a doubt, strengthen your relationships and provide you and your family with a sense of balance and *lagom*.

My mother is a master of *mys*. When you walk into my parent's house, you can literally feel the coziness. Part of this is because my mother loves to crank up the thermostat, so when you walk into the house, the heat wraps around you like a big warm hug. The lighting is always dim unless there is natural sunlight shining through. Dinners are eaten over candlelight; television watching is done the same way. For the longest while, I thought everyone enjoyed candlelit meals and cozy TV time!

To this day, I can count on one hand the number of times my mother has turned on the overhead kitchen lights—lights my family refers to as the "bright lights." The running joke in our household is that as long as there is enough light to see what we are eating, we are good. There have been times, however, when we have literally said to my mother, "Mom, we have to turn up the lights, we can't see our food!"

My family celebrates the wonderful benefits of *mys* by having an annual "*mys* night." This get-together consists of warm drinks (usually glögg, a type of Swedish mulled warm wine) being enjoyed around the outdoor fire pit, followed by a hearty dinner eaten in a very dimly lit dining room. The night concludes in the living room where we gather around the fireplace to play games and chat while cuddling under blankets.

I recommend trying this Swedish practice of finding joy and contentment in any situation for yourself! During your togetherness time, cuddle up in a warm blanket and enjoy a hot cup of coffee, tea, or hot cocoa. Add a roaring fire or some dimly lit candles to add to the cozy and relaxing experience. And remember, *mys* is about enjoying each other's company, so it can be done during any season, not just the winter months. Spend togetherness time by watching the sunset, cozying up on the couch, playing a board game, or enjoying a candlelit dinner together.

To create a warm, cozy, and relaxing atmosphere in your own space, try adding elements of *mys* throughout your home. Bring nature inside by decorating with natural materials, fresh flowers, and natural light, if possible. This doesn't need to be anything extravagant: just simple flowers to freshen up the space and add a bit of extra color and life.

Decorating with warm colors and comfortable fabrics is another way to make your home a place that's enjoyable for togetherness time. Swedes typically choose neutral colors: lots of shades of whites and subtle patterns, if any. Decor is meant to relax and refresh you, not overwhelm you. Create a sense of *mys* in your home to ensure a relaxing environment where togetherness time is the focus and strong family bonds are made and strengthened—all of which is essential to living a *lagom* lifestyle.

Mys Shopping Guide

Add these items to your shopping list to help create a *mys* atmosphere in your home.

- Blankets and soft woven throws in neutral colors
- Oversized pillows
- Candles
- Comfortable seating
- Cozy mugs
- Slippers
- In-season plants or flowers
- Yummy foods and beverages
- Decor made from natural elements

Fika
It's Not Just Coffee

Fika, literally translated, means coffee. Over the years, however, *fika* has become much more to Swedes than a word for coffee. Used to refer to a coffee break or breaking during the day to enjoy a cup of coffee and sweet treats, *fika* can be used as noun, a verb, or even an adjective. But while Sweden *does* have many delicious baked treats to enjoy, *fika* is more about the time spent together than the food which is served.

The key difference between American coffee breaks and *fika* is the all-important word, "enjoy." When you think of a coffee break in America, it's usually rushed, drunk as quickly as possible in order to get that jolt of caffeine into your body; it's seen as a way to be more productive and to get more done. *Fika*, on the other hand, is a mindful, thoughtful, and planned break in the day to slow down and appreciate the simple pleasures.

When visiting my *mormor* and *morfar*, they would often stop their day for what I now know was *fika*. They would pour a cup of coffee (from the percolator, as they never bought a coffee maker or Keurig) and cut a slice of homemade Swedish coffee bread or indulge in a few cookies together at the kitchen table. When I was younger, I just thought they both really liked sweets. I had no idea *fika* was a way to find balance during a busy day, a time to connect with loved ones, and a time to appreciate the little things. Looked at in this way, *fika* can be understood as a way of practicing *lagom* daily. Even the largest corporations in Sweden such as Volvo engage in the practice of *fika*. Production stops and all employees *fika*. What a great way to find balance during a busy and often hectic workday!

The main point of *fika* is to spend togetherness time with your family. It's about taking a break from the hustle and bustle of the day to reconnect. It shows your family that you are interested in learning about their day while showing the value of taking a break and focusing on the important parts of life. Remember, the endless tasks of daily work *can* wait ten minutes. *Fika* gives Swedes the much-needed benefit of regrouping, resetting, and recharging.

If you feel like you and your family need a way to find balance and recharge throughout the day, consider incorporating *fika* into your life. As with most Swedish traditions and concepts, it's okay to alter them to fit your needs.

For example, in our household, my mother would always have a snack ready for us after school. It was part of our routine: my mother would pick us up from school, we'd come home and have an after-school snack. We would often sit around the kitchen table and discuss our days while enjoying a tasty treat. Little did I know, this was *fika*. This time served as a way to come together as a family, even for just a little bit. I looked forward to sharing about my day and listening to my siblings discuss theirs. It was something I could look forward to during the day and something I could count on happening, a reassuring fixed point in my daily routine. Our own little family *fika* break provided stability, comfort, connection, and most importantly, balance.

As a practice that helps Swedes live a *lagom* lifestyle, here are some tips for your own *fika*!

- **Set a specific time of day to *fika*.** Scheduling a set time each day will help make *fika* a habit and part of your daily routine.

- **Embrace a *fika* and *lagom* mindset.** Keep things simple, focus on the present, and enjoy the break. Practice mindful eating by focusing on the taste, texture, and aroma of the coffee and treats. Refrain from multitasking and try not to think about what you should be doing, could be doing, would be doing, or what you must do later.

- **Adapt *fika* to fit best into your lifestyle.** Remember you can *fika* with all types of food and drinks. Get creative and choose tasty treats you and your family enjoy!

Fredagsmys
Swedish Friday Nights

The cultural importance of downtime and enjoying the simple things in life is of so much value to Swedes, they have even created specific days of the week to do exactly that. *Fredagsmys,* known to Swedes as "cozy Friday," is a portmanteau of *Fredags,* the Swedish word for Friday, and *mys*— literally meaning "cozy Friday." This concept allows togetherness to happen every Friday by giving your family a chance to spend time together and decompress at the end of each week.

Fredagsmys is something like watching television together wrapped in cozy blankets while enjoying good food. Swedes view this time as a way to connect with family members and typically encourage each family member, especially the youngest members, to take an active role in the planning of *fredagsmys* to make it even more of a family affair. For example, family members might take turns choosing which movies to watch or which yummy foods to eat. Feeling more involved in these family gatherings will only help maximize the positive benefits of togetherness time. This consistent time spent together becomes a routine that your entire family can count on, which leads to a greater connection. For this reason, *fredagsmys* is an easy, adaptable family time that can become a tradition with little work and planning required—a simple act with great reward!

I have fond memories of my family's "TV time." My family would make it a habit to watch television together not only on Fridays but every night from 8–9pm. We had specific shows we would watch every night while cuddling on the couch with our after-dinner treats and blankets. Even in the warmer months, we would still make our TV togetherness time cozy with comfortable pillows and lit candles all around our den. This was a special time we all looked forward to, gladly settling in after a day of school, work, or other family outings. In writing this book, I've come to realize how fortunate I am to have spent this daily time together with my family. It's something from our family that I'm proud to say continues to be passed down to the younger generations.

Fredagsmys and other *mys* or coziness time together is a way for you and your family to find balance throughout the days and weeks of life's busyness and distractions. Remember, incorporating *mys* into your family's life is about taking time together to enjoy the little things in life, surrounding yourself with loved ones and creating a cozy atmosphere at home.

Here are a few strategies to help you plan your own *fredagsmys* with your family and loved ones or by yourself:

Choose your menu. Keep it easy, simple, and fuss free!

Create your atmosphere. Lay out blankets and pillows and light a few candles.

Choose how to relax. Decide if you want to watch a show or movie, listen to music, read a book, play games, or chat with others.

Ett liv utan kärlek är
som ett år utan sommar.

"A LIFE WITHOUT LOVE IS LIKE
A YEAR WITHOUT SUMMER."

Swedish Traditions

A childhood is a manuscript that
we write our dreams on.

—Astrid Lindgren, Swedish author

Barn gör som du gör, inte som du säger.

—Swedish proverb

Meaning: Children do as you do,

not as you say.

By definition, a tradition is a belief or custom which is passed from one generation to another and which links us to those who came before. Traditions give us a sense of stability and help us connect with our roots, giving us insight into our own behaviors and reinforcing a sense of belonging. Traditions reflect a family's values and beliefs, and many children and family psychologists agree that traditions are an important part of childhood development. Traditional celebrations, for example, give both children and adults something to look forward to.

In essence, traditions build memories and memories are the unwritten record of our lives. Each new generation therefore has the ability, if not the responsibility, to create new traditions that reflect the lives we live today and communicate that information to those who will follow after us.

Let's take a look at a few of the traditions from the past that are celebrated by Swedish families today, including my own.

The Legend of Santa Lucia

There are many different versions of the story of Lucia which all intertwine to create a warm and joyous celebration. My tradition focuses on the story of a benevolent Lucia who brought food to the hungry villagers of Sweden during years of famine and was the bringer of light during the darkest days of winter. Lucia is derived from the Latin word *lux*, which means light.

Although the Feast of *Sankta* Lucia is not an official holiday in Sweden, it is celebrated on December 13th throughout the country, in churches, schools, professional buildings, hospitals, and shopping malls. The ceremony consists of a procession lead by Lucia dressed in a white cotton gown, red sash around her waist and a crown of lighted candles on her head. Her attendants, each holding a lit candle, follow behind her singing the song, "Santa Lucia." The words of the song speak to her benevolent nature and her ability to bring light and hope in the darkness of a cold and dreary Swedish winter:

Now in the winter night,
Good folk are waiting.
See now the maid of light,
Darkness abating.
Into our hearts she walks,
Telling her story,
Candles in shining crown
Lighting her glory.
Symbol of love sublime,
Moving o'er space and time,
Santa Lucia, Santa Lucia.
Into the winter night,
Come, maid of swing light,
Santa Lucia, Santa Lucia.
When on this earth she walked,
Bravely confessing,
All to the poor she gave,
All felt her blessing.
Ever her legend grew,
Spanning each ocean.
Light of the longest night,
Maid of devotion.

It is also a Swedish tradition that early on the morning of December 13th, the eldest daughter in the family, dressed as Lucia with her own crown of candles, brings coffee and special Christmas buns called *lussekatter* to her parents/other family members, all the while singing "Santa Lucia."

My memories of Santa Lucia Day are ones of early, dark, and cold winter mornings and the smell of "fresh" brewed coffee that we would reheat in the microwave. My mother would make the coffee the night before, since as kids we didn't know how to use the coffee maker. I would sneak a bite of the Swedish coffee bread, place lit candles on the serving tray, and follow my older sister (who would be playing the role of Saint Lucia) up the stairs and into my parent's bedroom. My brother would follow behind me, half asleep, singing with us.

My parents would pretend they were sleeping until they heard our soft voices singing *Santa Lucia*. After we were done singing, we would place the tray on the bed and climb onto it and enjoy the Swedish coffee bread with my parents. It was a cozy way to start the day with my family.

Giving your family the ability to reminisce about family traditions is invaluable. Fond memories such as these will stay with you for a lifetime and can help you find *lagom* during the more hectic and chaotic moments in life.

Memories of Santa Lucia

As told by my mother, Karen:

I was about five years old when I experienced my first Lucia pageant in my church, St. Mark's Lutheran Church in Bridgeport, Connecticut. The sanctuary was dark except for the candles in the window, and the church was full as I snuggled in between my mom and dad. Soon, the pianist began, and the sound of humming could be heard as the procession made its way up the stairs and into the narthex.

Then the doors swung open as Lucia and her attendants processed to the front of the church, singing Santa Lucia all the way. At the conclusion of the performance, coffee and Swedish baked goods were waiting for us in the fellowship hall. It's one of those warm childhood memories that stays with you for a lifetime.

In 1982, we moved to New Hampshire when my husband accepted the call to be the Pastor of Triumphant Cross Lutheran Church in Salem. I was surprised to learn that they did not celebrate Lucia Day, and as I wanted my children to experience the tradition that I had growing up, I set out to organize a pageant to do just that. We focused on Lucia's goodness and the light she brought into the world. To make the pageant relevant today, we included songs that the kids knew, such as *Twinkle, Twinkle, Little Star*. Others included *One Light,*

One Sun; another was *Light One Candle*; and of course, we added in a few Swedish songs like *Tre Pepparkaksgubbar,* to be sung as gingerbread kids passed out *pepparkakars* (a crispy Swedish cookie) to round out the performance. Afterwards, Swedish refreshments were served in the fellowship hall. This was another way to keep a tradition alive for the next generation.

I'm not sure why, but we didn't enact the morning ritual in my house when I was growing up. I guess some traditions just skip a generation, because my three kids would go on to treat my husband and I to coffee and Swedish coffee bread in the early morning hours of December 13th for years to come.

Today, my granddaughters dress in Lucia gowns and a crown of candles, climb the stairs early on December 13th to serve coffee and Swedish coffee bread to their parents.

God Jul
A Family Affair

God Jul translates to "good" or "merry Christmas" in Swedish. Today, most Swedes celebrate Christmas on December 24th, Christmas Eve, not December 25th. Many local customs have disappeared, yet each family celebrates in their own way, embracing their favorite traditions that best fit with their lifestyle.

By the time December 24th rolls around, the house has been thoroughly cleaned from top to bottom and decorated in accordance with the family's traditions. The food has been prepared and presents carefully arranged under the lighted tree. The *Jul Bord* or "Christmas table" is a buffet, featuring many different dishes including the Christmas ham, sausage (*korv*), pickled herring salad (*inlagd sill*), marinated salmon (*gralax*), rye bread (*vörtbörd*), boiled potatoes, meatballs, rice pudding, cheese, and a special fish dish called *lutefisk* which is a bit of an acquired taste! After dinner, Santa Claus, or *Jul Tomte*, arrives and is welcomed by the children as he hands out gifts to everyone.

The Christmas Tree
A Collection of
Treasured Memories

In years gone by, live trees covered with newly fallen snow were freshly cut and brought into the home. Smaller trees were selected because the farmhouses had low ceilings. The first Swedish Christmas trees were decorated with lit candles, fruits, and candy. Later on, homemade ornaments of straw and wood were added to the collection.

Decorating the Christmas tree was and remains a family affair in our household. It's something my siblings and I looked forward to every year, as it represented the beginning of the Christmas season. Before we began decorating the tree, I can remember taking out all the ornaments from their boxes and unwrapping them from their protective paper towels. Today, my parents have upgraded from paper towels to proper ornament storage boxes—I'm pretty sure we can attribute that to my father's passion for *Döstädning*.

In the boxes, we would find all of our personalized ornaments as well as handcrafted ornaments we had made in years past. (It was a known rule that personalized ornaments were only allowed to be hung by the person whose name was on it or who had made that specific ornament.) Finding the perfect spot to hang our ornaments was a task in itself. My siblings and I swear, to this day, that my father would sneak down to the living room after we went to bed and reposition the ornaments so that tree looked better and more balanced. Perhaps my father was just trying to create a *lagom Jul* tree.

While decorating the tree, we would be playing Christmas music and enjoying warm, cozy snacks. We would take turns showing the ornaments we had unwrapped to others while recounting stories and memories that ornament inspired. When you placed "your" ornaments on the tree, it offered a way to connect with the past as well as provide a sense of belonging and a sense of self.

Our Swedish Christmas tree was adorned with traditional Swedish ornaments: beautifully made straw and wooden Christmas goats, Dala horses, snowflakes, and *Jültomten* trimmed our tree. When I was younger, I never understood why my parents wouldn't let us have flashy tinsel or colored lights, but looking back on it now, I am extremely grateful for the meaningful Christmas tree my parents created every year for us. The Swedish Christmas tree is a visual representation of family connection and cohesion: a perfect balance of each individual family member and their individual memories, displayed together in one spot.

Karen's Christmas Memories

Our Christmas tree today embraces the past and celebrates the present. There are straw goats, angels, and heart-shaped ornaments, *Jul Tomtes*, hand-painted Dala horses, and shiny paper cut-out decorations. Some were bought in specialty Swedish shops in Connecticut and New Hampshire; others were gifts from relatives living in Sweden. There are a number of homemade salt dough ornaments of wreaths, *Jul Tomtes*, and gingerbread people, glazed and painted by my children.

Milestones, special occasions, and personal interests are also on display, each one carefully hung on just the right branch. (Although, it really didn't matter, as when everyone was tucked in for the night, my husband would rearrange the ornaments to his satisfaction.) There are baby's first Christmases; pianos, guitars and trumpets for the music lovers; and baseballs and gloves, skis, and sailboats for the sport enthusiasts in the family.

A fire engine reminds our family of when my son was a firefighter, a plane for when he started flying, and a shiny, golden Starbuck's coffee mug (of all things) to remind us of our trip to Philadelphia for a wedding. Sand, beach chairs, and palm trees remind us of our vacations to the island of St. John.

Even with all the presents, the food, the tree, and the decorations, the most important part of Christmas is...togetherness. Being together, remembering the past, celebrating the present, making new traditions, and looking forward to what the future holds is what Christmas is all about for our family—enjoying our Swedish heritage. What a wonderful way to find *lagom* during the busy holiday season!

Of course, today our tree is artificial, and Hallmark provides ornaments and decorations, but that's okay. The traditions are still alive and each year when Christmas is over, the ornaments from the past are carefully stored in our attic alongside our present-day decorations. As our life situations change, so do the ways in which we celebrate. We do what is necessary to capture the balance that is essential for a healthy, happy life. Or, as the Swedes say: *lagom.*

Is It Easter or Halloween?

Barnaminnet är långt.

—Swedish proverb translated as,
"Childhood memories last long."

Childhood memories, as told by my mother, Karen:

As Sweden is more of a secular country, Easter is less a religious celebration and more of a tradition that provides an opportunity to spend time with family. It is especially designed to be a delightful experience for children. It is the first long weekend after winter, so families travel to their summer homes in the south and ski cabins in the north and continue to make lasting memories.

In fact, Sweden's celebration of Easter looks more like America's Halloween. In Sweden today, both boys and girls dress up as witches wearing head scarves, long skirts, and painted faces. They go house to house giving their neighbors home-made drawings, paintings, and cards. In return, they receive candy. Later, they are given large decorative eggs filled with candy.

Our family has not continued this Easter walk practice; however, we do enjoy the tradition of the *Paskris,* or Easter Tree. The tree is usually made from birch or willow twigs decorated with colored feathers and hand-painted eggs. The Easter Tree is yet another way to bring nature into our home to celebrate spring.

Once again, this tradition skipped a genera-tion. We did not have an Easter Tree when I was growing up. However, the tradition was revived with my children and now with my granddaugh-ters. It's another opportunity to spend time together. We pick birch twigs from the trees in our backyard, place them in a tall, sturdy crystal vase and then carefully hang the crafted eggs and feathers on the branches. Over the years, we've added store-bought paper eggs.

Writing this, I've realized there are some traditions (such as celebrating *Santa Lucia* at home, creating an Easter Tree, making *glögg* and others) that were not part of my household growing up. I believe the reason for this was because my mother was so intent on becoming Americanized that she purposely shed her Swedish traditions. After all, she was busy attending night school to learn English, taking driving lessons, and studying for her citizenship test. It's because of the absence of these customs in my childhood that I made every effort to make sure my kids didn't miss out on the traditions that have since influenced and shaped their lives.

To ensure family togetherness time, make it a goal of yours to start a new family tradition. Over ten years ago, I began what is now known in our family as the Fall Festival of Family Fun. It's a day filled with fun family time. We play games in the backyard while enjoying fall-themed food and drinks and end the night around the firepit. This tradition is something we all look forward to and hope to continue for generations to come. Choose a tradition that is a good fit for you and your family. The Swedish secret to a *lagom* life, one filled with balance, is most definitely the time spent with loved ones.

Swedish Cooking

Låt maten tysta munnen.

—Swedish proverb
Meaning: Let the food silence the mouth.

Like traditions, recipes have a way of carrying on the memories and stories of the past. Family recipes, for example, are a way to connect to past and present generations and to find comfort and familiarity in an ever-changing world. Family recipes are often passed down through generations, while the tradition of cooking or baking together with family often lends itself to sharing stories of the past while planning for the future.

When you think about Swedish food, the first item that usually comes to mind for many is the very famous Swedish meatball. The second is typically the Swedish *smörgåsbord*, alongside lesser-known Swedish delicacies like pickled herring (which is actually pretty good), Jansson's temptation (which is basically a potato casserole), and rice pudding topped with lingonberries. The typical Swedish diet is composed mostly of fish, whole grains, lean proteins, hearty vegetables, berries, and fermented dairy. I would consider that a well-balanced diet—another boon for living a *lagom* life. If that doesn't sound appealing to you, don't worry; the *lagom* lifestyle is all about finding the right balance for you and your family.

Truth be told, many of my family's Swedish recipes have been altered over the years. The great thing about family recipes is that you can change them to fit your family's current needs. See? Even recipes can be *lagom*! For example, while traditional Swedish meatballs call for a mixture of pork, veal, and beef, my mother makes hers with ground turkey meat, as my family members aren't big red meat eaters. I make my Swedish meatballs with plant-based ingredients since half of my family are pescatarians. And after all, it's the traditional Swedish spices that make any type of meatball delicious!

After my *mormor* died in 2020, we tried to replicate many of her recipes. We were fortunate enough to have saved her handwritten recipe cards, which we later turned into a printed photo recipe book. Having her handwriting and seeing the food and drink stains on the recipe cards makes us feel connected to her, which in turn makes baking these family recipes even more special and meaningful.

Little did we know, until trying to recreate these recipes ourselves, is that my *mormor's* measurements were often…lacking. My sister and I would then consult with my mother and ask how much butter or cardamom was needed, as my *mormor* just wrote "a dash" or "a scant." My mother would nod as if she knew exactly how much my *mormor's* recipe was calling for and respond with, "Until it seems right." If that's not baking with *lagom*, I don't know what is.

Making Swedish coffee bread is another staple in any Swedish household. It's a long process but definitely worth it. It's a family affair as we all take turns braiding the dough and sprinkling on the *pärlsocker* (pearl sugar). The smell of cardamom fills the kitchen, and when the bread comes out of the oven, everyone delights in the wonderful and delicious masterpiece.

Then there are *pepparkakor* cookies, which are similar to gingersnaps, but much less gingery. If you could taste Christmas, it would taste like Swedish *pepparkakor*. They, too, are a labor of love. I grew up with homemade *pepparkakor* made by my *mormor*. They were delicious, with just the perfect thinness—which anyone who has attempted to make these cookies knows is no easy feat. Legend says if you make a wish while holding the *pepparkakor* in the palm of your hand, if you lightly tap it and it breaks into three pieces, your wish will come true. Both the wonderful balance of spices and the hope of your wish coming true makes for wonderful holiday *lagom*.

Sorry mom, but I couldn't write about *pepparkakors* and not include this memory. My most memorable experience with *pepparkakors* came when I was about ten years old. My mother, sister, brother, and I were all standing around the kitchen table getting ready to roll out the *pepparkakor* dough. We had all the cookie cutters out and ready to go. There was a fine selection, too: we had a few in the shape of Dala horses, hearts, and stars. My mother helped us roll out our section of the dough and once that was done, we were ready to start pressing down the cookie cutters.

So far, so good. All the cookies were pressed and ready to be transported to the cookie sheet. But the first Dala horse didn't make it. Then, neither did the second one, or the third one, or the hearts or any of the stars. The dough was so thin it was nearly impossible to pick them up with the spatula we had without damaging them. We lost a lot of Dala horse legs that day. We tried over and over and over again, until finally my mother had had enough and said, "Just forget it, go outside and play, we will buy some *pepparkakor* cookies!" That was the last time my mother ever tried to make *pepparkakor* cookies with us. Fast forward about 30 years and our family *pepparkakors* are back to being homemade, thanks to my oldest niece, Helena!

One of my family's favorite and most often made Swedish recipes is without a doubt *glögg*.

Even my British father is a huge fan of *glögg*. Some may say it's an acquired taste, but to us Swedes, it's *mys* in a mug! *Glögg* is most easily described as a mulled wine, but with a lot of extra booze added to the mix. Everyone's family recipe is a little different, as ours does not contain the traditional almonds, since my father is allergic, or raisins. (I'm not sure why we don't add raisins; I guess my mother just never cared for them.) *Glögg* is a wonderful mixture of oranges, lemons, cloves, cardamom, cinnamon, and ginger combined with port wine, a sweet white wine, brandy, vodka, and sugar.

Swedes believe *glögg* to be more than just a delicious drink that helps keep you warm throughout the winter. It is said that *glögg* has medicinal purposes. If you aren't feeling well, a small glass of *glögg* will do the trick and have you feeling better in no time. I swear it works! I speak from experience; nothing clears out your sinuses better than a glass of *glögg*.

The point is, it doesn't matter if your family recipes come out perfectly or are exactly the way your *mormor* made them. It's about spending time together with your family and finding the right balance. The Swedes know the secret to happiness isn't about perfection, it's about *lagom*.

To this day when I think about my *mormor's* spice cake, I can smell it as if it were on a plate in front of me. The strong and warm aroma of cloves will forever remind me of my *mormor*. I may be biased, but she made the best spice cake, spritz cookies, and Swedish cinnamon buns. (My mother makes the best Swedish coffee bread.)

One of my most favorite holiday traditions is still baking family recipes with my mother, sister, and nieces. Every year we make Swedish coffee bread, spice cake, *pepparkakor* cookies, and *glögg*. It wouldn't be Christmas without these essential sweet treats. We start early in December so that we can have Swedish coffee bread on the morning of Santa Lucia Day and *glögg* to drink throughout the cold winter months.

Creating your own traditions. Even if you aren't Swedish, you can incorporate your own traditions into your life. Below are a few ideas to help get your started.

Choose an activity or area of interest that you or your family enjoy. Maybe it's planning an annual summer hike, or trip to the beach. Perhaps you would like to start creating a ritual of always enjoying the same menu for certain holidays or watching the same Christmas movies.

Pass these traditions down to other generations or even your friend group. Monthly get-togethers to catch up with one another or signing up for the same road race are other ways to stay connected.

Traditions can also be applied to individuals. Reading the same book once a year or going to the beach every year on the first day of summer can be yearly outings you look forward to doing.

Set a personal goal this year to create a new tradition. The possibilities are endless, so have fun thinking up new ways of spending time with loved ones or enjoying time for yourself.

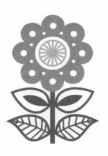

The Importance of Living Lagom

Swedish Living During Stressful Times

During the height of the 2020 global pandemic, we learned firsthand the difficulties of combating social isolation. In that time of uncertainly, high anxiety, and separation, the benefits of a *lagom* lifestyle were appreciated like never before.

While no amount of *lagom* lifestyle habits could have prevented a disaster of that scale, the art of Swedish living and finding joy in just enough helped loved ones find balance and relief in an unpredictable time. Creating a family unit that practices *lagom* living while celebrating annual traditions such as cozy Friday nights or daily *fika* increases feelings of belonging and decreases the negative effects of loneliness. Creating a sense of *mys* in your home and an environment where family togetherness and con-nectedness is a priority brings about balanced

living. Remember, meaningful and close relationships directly impact your sense of belonging,
something I'm sure everyone could use more of,
especially in unsettled situations.

The point is that the stronger your bonds are,
forged through time spent together meaning-
fully and intentionally, the better able you and
everyone connected to you are to cope with
unexpected hardships.

During COVID, my family and I lived a lifestyle
true to our Swedish roots. Time spent in nature
increased; a slower-paced life filled with more
lagom was easier to achieve; *mys* nights spent
around fire pits or TV watching with dimly lit candles all around became the norm. More evenings
were spent outside watching the sunset while
playing board games or just engaging in conver-
sation. Family meals occurred more often than just
breakfast and dinner and everyone gained a new
appreciation for the simpler things in life. Simply
put, COVID allowed for more family togetherness

time and more opportunities to experience things together.

Now, by no means am I discounting the negative impact of COVID. I would obviously never wish for another pandemic or for anyone to experience the significant loss that was associated with the coronavirus. However, when situations are out of your control, it's important to remember to focus only on what *is* within your control. This mindset will help you and your family find *lagom*.

Swedish Living Successes

Over the years, there have been many notable accomplishments and innovations created by great Swedish thinkers! These Swedes were able to successfully accomplish their goals while maintaining a *lagom* lifestyle. Such success stories include the first implantable pacemaker (developed by Rune Elmquist in 1958), Electrolux household appliances, the "monkey wrench," the three-point seatbelt, the zipper, the walker, H&M Fashion, Spotify, Volvo, the Nobel Peace Prize (named after Alan Noble, the Swede responsible for the creation of dynamite), and perhaps the most well-known Swedish company, IKEA.

These success stories are living proof that personal balance and professional success are possible…and that we would all be better off living like the Swedes! Finding joy in just enough can be mastered by all and the benefits of *lagom* will positively impact you and your family for generations to come.

How to Act Like a Swede

Respect personal space. Don't stand too close or hug without being invited to do so. Swedish people are not overly friendly to strangers and value their independence and personal space. Only expect hugs once you have become a member of someone's inner circle.

Take off your shoes. Outdoor shoes are never—and I mean *never*—worn inside. Even the thought of someone wearing outdoor shoes in a bedroom makes me cringe. At my house, we have outdoor shoes and indoor shoes, and ne'er the twain shall meet.

Be punctual. Swedes are known for being on time and they do not appreciate when others are late. Swedish people value and respect the time of others. Whether it be a business meeting, midday *fika*, or family movie nights, events begin on time.

Be environmentally conscious. Sustainability and eco-friendliness are strongly emphasized throughout Swedish culture. Sweden was the first country to pass an environmental protection act in 1967 and hosted the first UN conference on the global environment in 1972.

Don't be loud. Swedes are considered to be a relatively quiet people. They don't often talk loudly nor are they overly expressive, especially in public. Swedes, by nature, are fairly calm, reserved, and even-tempered. Unfortunately, this is sometimes construed as snobbery or off-putting, which couldn't be further from the truth. Swedes don't think they are better than others; they are just content and confident in their silence.

Don't be overly familiar. Swedes do not engage in small talk. They find small talk to be a waste of time and energy and would rather engage in meaningful conversations with familiar people. Swedes believe less is more when it comes to conversing. They are focused and like to get to the point quickly. Remember, time is precious... so why waste it talking about insignificant pleasantries?

Always leave the last piece. If you are sharing snacks with Swedes, you will quickly notice no one takes the last piece of food. Swedes view doing so as rude, selfish, and inconsiderate. Much discussion is had over who should take the last piece. It is only after everyone has okay-ed it that someone is allowed to enjoy the last bit of food.

*De som önskar att sjunga
hittar alltid en låt.*

"THOSE WHO WISH TO SING,
ALWAYS FIND A SONG."

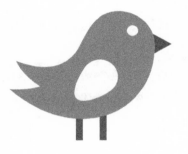

Enjoy Your Journey

It goes without saying that it's easier to live *lagom* in its country of origin. Sweden has specific governmental and federal policies in place that make it easier to find balance and create a *lagom* life. For example, Sweden provides families with a significantly greater amount of parental leave than in the United States, with a full year of maternal and parental leave being common. This naturally affords families the opportunity to spend more time together and find balance with one another. Imagine all the benefits you and your family would experience if you were able to spend more time together living the *lagom* life!

But despite this lack of "natural advantages," living a life of *lagom* is still very possible, and well worth striving for. Wholeheartedly believing in the benefits of a Swedish lifestyle and the practice of *lagom* helps foster togetherness time, creating lasting memories and family traditions that will be passed down from you to your child and beyond. It's this very special time together that shows your family that everyone is invested in each other's lives and appreciates the time spent with one another. Incorporating these Swedish philosophies into your own family life, regardless of whether you were born a Swede or not, will create a family lifestyle filled with *lagom*, timeless traditions, and togetherness—all qualities that represent a happy, healthy, and balanced life.

I am very grateful that my parents (my father openly adopted the Swedish way of life, while sprinkling a bit of his British influence too) passed along these very simple, yet very impactful ways of living. If you yourself are not lucky enough to have Swedish heritage, you can still embrace and practice the basic ways of living like a Swede. These philosophies and overall mindsets will help you enjoy life and everyone in it.

We hope you have enjoyed this book as much as we enjoyed writing it together. Remember, *lagom* is all about finding "just the right amount" and living a balanced life. Tailor the traditions, routines and lifestyle habits found in this book to best fit your needs and your family's needs. Take time to appreciate the little things in life, surround yourself with family and loved ones, continue family traditions, embrace the outdoors, and don't forget to clean!

Tack sä mycket!
Thank you!

Efter regn

kommer solsken.

"AFTER RAIN COMES SUNSHINE."

About the Authors

Kortney Yasenka is a licensed clinical mental health counselor with a Masters in Counseling Psychology with a concentration in Health Psychology from Northeastern University. Kortney has worked in community mental health, school systems, and private practice. Thanks to her mother being 100% Swedish, the values of a Swedish lifestyle were embedded into her daily living. Kortney embraces the *lagom* lifestyle and is an advocate for everyone to learn how to live like a Swede. In her free time she enjoys running, spending time with family, cheering on the Cleveland Guardians and Cleveland Browns, and vacationing on the beautiful island of St. John.

Karen Johnson Yasenka grew up in Fairfield, CT, surrounded by Swedish friends and family. Swedish on both sides of her heritage, her mother immigrated to America in 1948 from Avesta, Sweden. In keeping with the Swedish commitment to community involvement, Karen has advocated for quality education (not just for her children, but for all children) and has organized fundraisers for local non-profits supporting the homeless and the elderly. She lives in New Hampshire with her husband and has three adult children. In her spare time, Karen enjoys visits to the Maine coast, playing the piano, and spending time with family, especially her granddaughters, Helena and Isla.

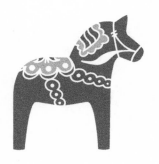

Bibliography

1. Xygalatas, D. Ritual: How Seemingly Senseless Acts Make Life Worth Living. Little Brown Spark, 2022.

2. www.psychologytoday.com/us/basics/emotion-regulation

3. Eisenberg N, Sadovsky A, Spinrad TL. Associations of emotion-related regulation with language skills, emotion knowledge, and academic outcomes. New Dir Child Adolesc Dev. 2005 Fall;(109):109-18.

4. www.nytimes.com/2023/01/03/well/live/awe-wonder-dacher-keltner.html

5. Jimenez MP, DeVille NV, Elliott EG, Schiff JE, Wilt GE, Hart JE, James P. Associations between Nature Exposure and Health: A Review of the Evidence. Int J Environ Res Public Health. 2021 Apr 30;18(9):4790.

6. Mead MN. Benefits of sunlight: a bright spot for human health. Environ Health Perspect. 2008 Apr;116(4):A160-7.

7. doi.org/10.1016/j.ufug.2015.02.006

8. journals.sagepub.com/doi/pdf/10.1177/147470490500300109

9. Saxbe D, Repetti RL. For better or worse? Coregulation of couples' cortisol levels and mood states. J Pers Soc Psychol. 2010 Jan;98(1):92-103.

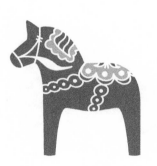